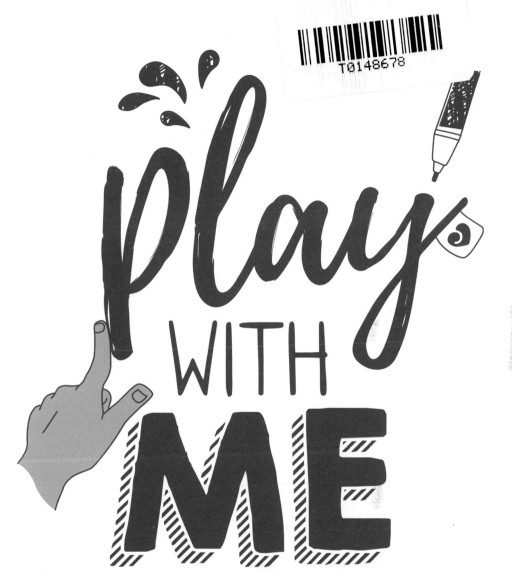

Play WITH ME

AN ACTIVITY BOOK FOR ADULTS

ICE HOUSE BOOKS

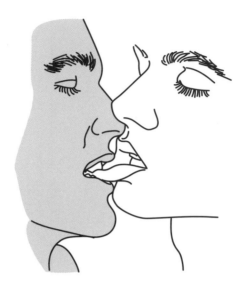

 Published by Ice House Books

Designed & illustrated by Amy McHugh

Ice House Books is an imprint of Half Moon Bay Limited
The Ice House, 124 Walcot Street, Bath, BA1 5BG
www.icehousebooks.co.uk

ISBN 978-1-913308-06-3

Printed in China

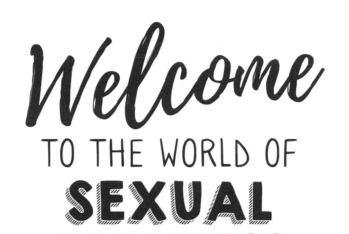

Welcome
TO THE WORLD OF
SEXUAL HAPPINESS

Lovehoney believes in making sex fun and fulfilling
for everyone. The art of play helps partners learn more about
their bodies, desires and needs in the bedroom. This book
explores the playful side of sexual activity and, by completing
the activities, puzzles and games with your partner, you can
discover more about each other than you ever knew before.
Or, of course, you can spend some alone time with this book.
The activities inside might prompt you to share your secret
fantasies, say things out loud that you might have been
too shy to say before, and open yourselves up
to fun in the bedroom – and beyond...

Safety & CONSENT

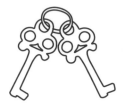

Firstly, just a few words about any sexual activities you enjoy while completing this book.

It's important to remember that any role-play scenarios in this book are complete fantasy, only to be acted out by those in trusting relationships. Never try them with anyone you're not already in a comfortable sexual relationship with.

Before embarking on any sort of BDSM journey (Bondage, Domination/Discipline, Sadism/ Submission, Masochism), there are some rules you must follow to

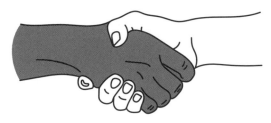

ensure everything is safe and everyone involved is having fun. At no point should bondage put either person at risk of injury. If something is distractingly painful or uncomfortable, stop immediately, and never leave a restrained person unattended.

Ensure that everyone involved is of sound mind. Never explore bondage or spanking while under the influence of drugs or alcohol.

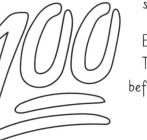

Everything you do together should be 100% consensual. To ensure this is the case, agree a safe word or action before you play. Safe words or actions are used by partners to indicate that they want play to stop immediately.

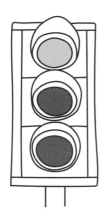

Choose a word that is short and easy to remember before play, or try the popular 'traffic light' system, where 'red' means stop, 'amber' means take it easy and 'green' means go on. If you use a gag, you'll need to agree a safe action instead. Clicking fingers, tapping a hard surface three times or opening and closing your hands repeatedly are popular choices. Avoid using household items that require a knot for first-time bondage. Keep a pair of specially designed safety scissors nearby just in case.

Only share personal photographs or videos of yourself with someone you completely trust. Remember once they are out in the world it's hard to get them back.

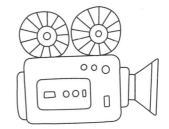

Remember these points and let the fun begin!

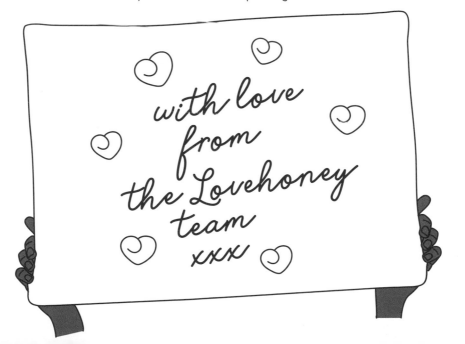

with love from the Lovehoney team xxx

SEARCH FOR SATISFACTION

Can you find these sexy words in the grid?

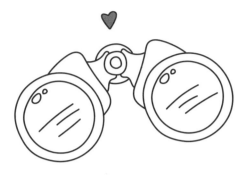

- ☐ BONDAGE
- ☐ BREASTS
- ☐ CLIMAX
- ☐ COME
- ☐ DOMINATION

- ☐ FINGERS
- ☐ G-SPOT
- ☐ MASSAGE
- ☐ MOUTH
- ☐ NIPPLES

- ☐ ORAL
- ☐ ORGASM
- ☐ PENIS
- ☐ PERMISSION
- ☐ PUNISH

- ☐ RESTRAINTS
- ☐ SEX
- ☐ SPANK
- ☐ SUBMISSION
- ☐ VIBRATOR

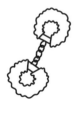

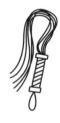

E	U	H	E	F	X	N	K	N	A	P	S
H	R	T	I	I	X	A	M	I	L	C	E
E	D	U	T	G	T	A	O	P	P	G	I
N	R	O	R	D	E	H	D	P	E	S	O
L	Y	M	M	O	C	G	A	L	R	P	X
P	M	S	H	I	T	I	A	E	M	O	M
E	S	T	N	S	N	A	G	S	I	T	X
N	A	S	T	N	I	A	R	T	S	E	R
I	G	A	I	L	D	N	T	B	S	A	E
S	R	E	G	N	I	F	U	I	I	E	M
D	O	R	O	R	A	L	N	P	O	V	O
S	U	B	M	I	S	S	I	O	N	N	C

Sex Sketch

Draw your ideal sexual activity on this page.

Then show your partner and see if you can bring it to life.

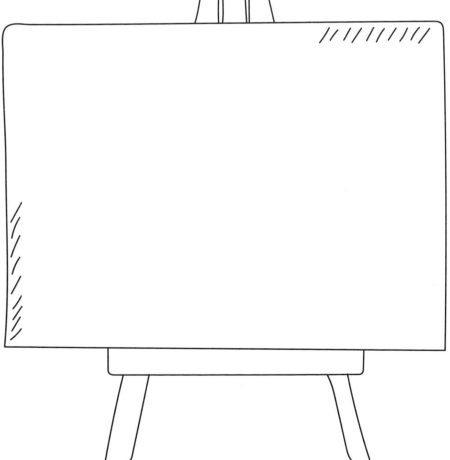

G-SPOT THE DIFFERENCE
P-SPOT THE DIFFERENCE

Can you find 8 differences between these two images?
Circle the changes in the second picture.

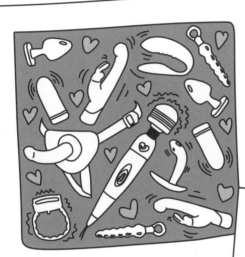

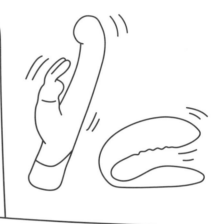

#PLEASURE TOWN

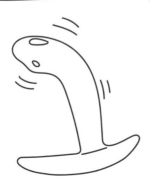

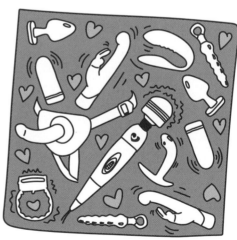

#PLEASURE TOWN

Position Yourself

Draw a sexual position you'd like to try...

I'M HARD

Can you conquer this hard codeword grid? Work out which letter matches which number and fill in the sexual positions. We've given one letter to get you started.

HOLD TIGHT

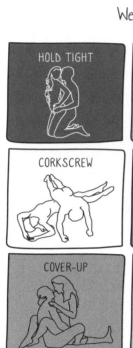

FISHBONE

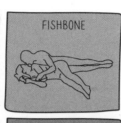

LOVE SEAT

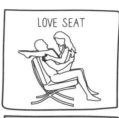

STAND AND DELIVER

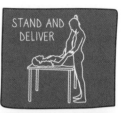

CORKSCREW

GIDDY-UP

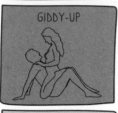

LUSTY LEAN

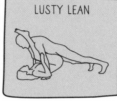

TABLE TOP

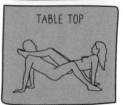

COVER-UP

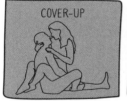

FLYING HIGH

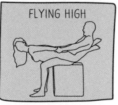

OPEN SESAME

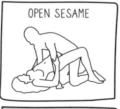

SEE-SAW

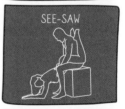

DANCER

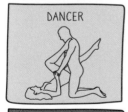

ROCK CHICK

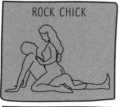

ROCK AND LOCK

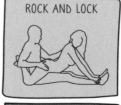

WHEELBARROW

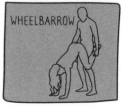

DOGGY STYLE

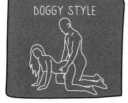

SEXY YOGA

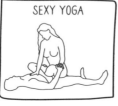

SEXY SPOON

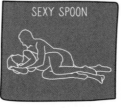

X-RATED

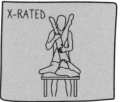

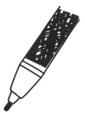

1	2	3	4	5	6	7	8	9	10	11	12	13

14	15	16	17	18	19	20	21	22	23	24	25	26
							P					

Dirty Secrets

Crack the code to work out these talking-dirty phrases.
Then why not try using them on your partner tonight?
Several letters are there to get you started.
See if you can fill in the rest.

A	B	C	D	E	F	G	H	I	J	K	L	M
9				8			3	15				

N	O	P	Q	R	S	T	U	V	W	X	Y	Z
	11				13	6		16			5	

1)

15		16	9	18	13		13	11		13	9	21	13	8		5	11	6

2)

16	3	8	1	8		20	11		5	11	6		16	9	18	13

14	8		13	11		12	11	14	8

3)

15		16	9	18	13		13	11		3	8	9	1

5	11	6		4	8	24

4)

24	8	13		11	18		5	11	6	1		10	18	8	8	21

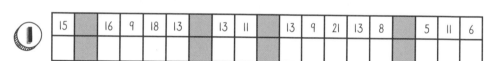

5.

4	8	18	20		11	26	8	1		15		9	14		24	11	15	18	24

13	11		21	17	9	18	10		5	11	6

6.

16	9	13	12	3		16	3	15	7	8		15		13	11	6	12	3

14	5	21	8	7	2

7.

15		16	9	18	13		5	11	6		13	11		2	*	12	10

14	5		14	11	6	13	3

8.

9	1	8		5	11	6		1	8	9	20	5		13	11

12	11	14	8		9	24	9	15	18		2	11	1		14	8

9.

7	8	13	21		16	9	13	12	3		17	11	1	18

13	11	24	8	13	3	8	1

10.

5	11	6		7	11	11	10		21	8	22	5		16	3	8	18

5	11	6		24	11		20	11	16	18		11	18		14	8

13

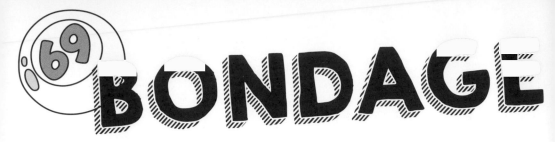

BONDAGE

Remove your lover's shirt or top, but leave it on their arms. Grab the fabric around their wrists to create a restraint.

Tie your partner's wrists together and tell them you're going to pleasure them, but they aren't allowed to make a noise.

Tie your lover's hands to the head of the bed then kneel over them and tell them to pleasure you with their mouth for as long as you desire.

For the next 5 minutes, your partner is your slave. They must do what you tell them, or they will be punished.

Think about an outfit your partner wears that really turns you on. Tell them to wear it and only you can undress them.

Bind your partner's arms above their head and play with their nipples. Try gentle tweaking, pinching, licking and even nibbling – but start gently!

Blindfold your partner and tell them to undress you, using just their sense of touch.

Tie your lover's hands in front of them, then tell them to kneel on the floor and pleasure you with their tongue.

Sit your lover in a chair and bind their hands behind it. Then either bring them to climax with your mouth, or tease them until they beg to be released.

Blindfold your lover. Select three items of food and feed them to your partner. Ask them to guess what they're tasting, and if they get it wrong, punish them.

Tie your partner's ankles and wrists. Then sit in a position where they can clearly see you, and make them watch you play with yourself.

Blindfold your partner and instruct them to touch themselves. Just before they climax, tell them to stop.

Get a little nibbly with your lover. Gently bite their lip as you kiss them, then bite their neck, their earlobes and the insides of their thighs.

Tie your lover's hands above their head with them lying on their front. Gently run the tips of your nails across their bare skin, all over their body.

Blindfold your lover and then, with them on the bottom, perform oral sex in the 69 position until you're close to climaxing, then stop.

Use a tie or scarf to gag your lover, and then tie their hands above their head. Pleasure them any way that you want and encourage them to be as loud as they can through the gag.

BINGO

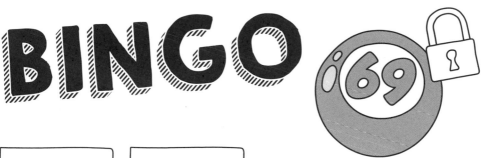

Tell your partner to close their eyes and place their own finger randomly on these pages. Do the activity together and cross it out on the grid.

Keep going until you've made a line horizontally or vertically.

Tell your lover to kneel, then blindfold them and tie their ankles and wrists. Gently tease them using any method of your choosing.

Grab a clothes peg and experiment with pinching areas of your lover's skin. Start with their finger tips, then the toes. If they enjoy it, progress to more sensitive areas.*

Bind your lover's wrists and ankles while they're lying on their back. Now, pop an ice cube in your mouth and kiss your partner on their most sensitive parts.

Pick an outfit that makes you feel sexy and powerful and tell your partner to dress you. Now tie them up and perform a sultry striptease.

Tell your lover to get on all fours. Stand behind them and spank them gently on the bottom ten times with the back of a hairbrush, and ask them to say 'thank you' after each strike.

Using any method of your choosing, bring your partner almost to the point of climax, then stop. Only continue when they beg you to carry on.

Tell your partner a name or word you would like to be called during sex or foreplay. For the rest of the game, they must refer to you only by this, and not your given name.

Tie your partner's hands somewhere high above their head while they're standing up. Now perform oral sex on them.

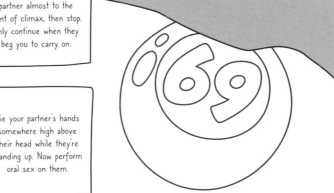

*Never leave a peg in place for longer than 10 minutes.

COLOUR ME SEXY

Colour in these sexual positions.

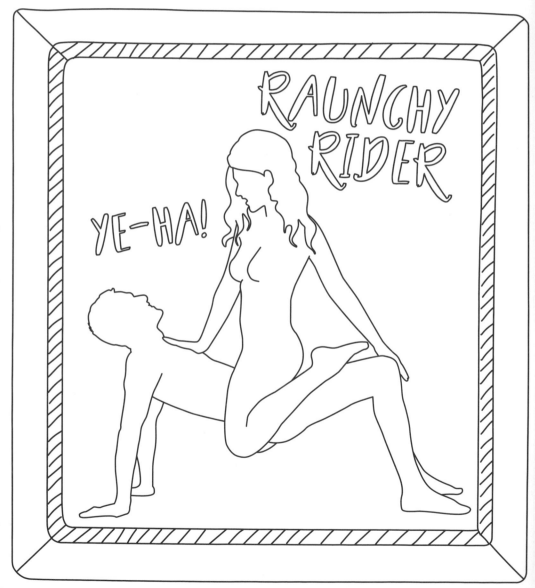

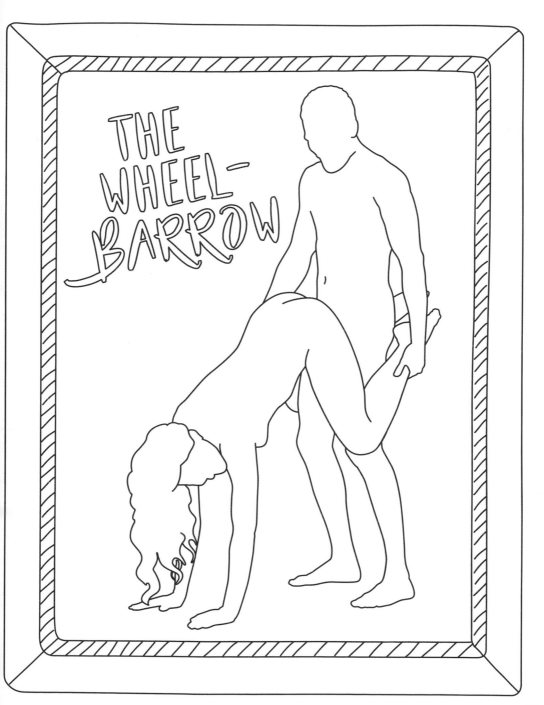

Hotword Crosswords

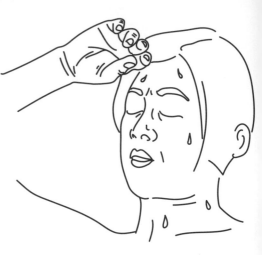

Phew... it's getting hot in here! Complete this crossword before all hell breaks loose! Unless you want it to...

ACROSS

3. To ask desperately for something. (3)
4. To pass the tongue over a surface. (4)
5. To make (someone) suffer for bad behaviour. (6)
7. To move toward someone or something, or to have an orgasm. (4)
8. To move continuously and rapidly to and fro, or pulsate (like a sex toy). (7)
10. To put your hand, fingers, etc. on someone or something. (5)
11. Intercourse or lovemaking. (3)
13. To cover the eyes of a person with a piece of cloth. (9)
14. To tie or wrap something with rope, string, etc. (4)
16. A planned occasion with your partner. (4)
18. The part of the body used for kissing. (5)
19. The sexual practice that involves being restrained (or restraining your partner). (7)

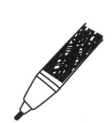

DOWN

1. One of the pieces that forms a bird's plumage – good for tickling. (7)
2. One of the two darker circles on the chest that are extra-sensitive and can be stimulated with suckers or clamps. (6)
6. Used to hold something or someone in place. (10)
9. To press down on (someone or something) with the teeth. (4)
12. The most popular _____ for sex is missionary. (8)
13. A room used for sleeping and other pleasurable things. (7)
15. To go down into a position where one or both knees are on the ground. (5)
17. To hit someone on the buttocks with your hand as a form of punishment. (5)

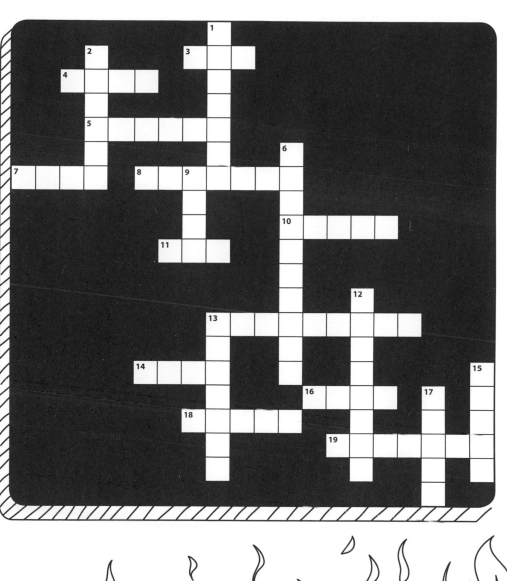

LET'S GET QUIZ-ICAL

Quiz your partner with these questions to find out more about their sexual interests. You might learn something you didn't already know. Then answer them for yourself and share with your partner.

1. Which of these appeals to you the most?

a) being restrained during sex
b) having sex outdoors
c) being watched while we have sex

2. During sex, would you rather I call you...

a) Sir or Madam
b) naughty
c) a different name to your own

3. Which of these places would you most like to receive oral sex?

a) in a lift
b) in the woods with nobody around
c) in the kitchen
d) in the bedroom
e) in a tent

4. Which of these parts of your body do you like me to touch the most?

a) your lips
b) your bottom
c) your waist
d) your breasts / chest
e) your feet

5. What would you like me to wear in the bedroom?

a) nothing
b) sexy lingerie
c) office clothes you can strip off
d) nothing but socks
e) pyjamas

6. When do you most like to have sex?

a) when we first wake up
b) just before we go to sleep
c) when we get home from work
d) in the afternoon (if we're not at work!)

7. Which position do you like the most?

a) missionary – on top
b) missionary – underneath
c) doggy style
d) standing up
e) 69
f) other ....

8. Which of these role-play scenarios would you most like to act out?

a) Firefighter – one of us called for the fire service and the other is a rather sexy firefighter...
b) Flight Attendant & Passenger – join the Mile High Club!
c) Alien & Earthling – show them the way of your species...
d) Travelling Strangers – we're both on a business trip, we've never met before...

9. What type of porn would you like to watch with me?

a) group sex
b) women together
c) men together
d) animation
e) bondage
f) none – let's make our own
g) I would rather read a sexy story

10. Which of these would you like to eat or lick off my body?

a) whipped cream
b) chocolate mousse
c) strawberries
d) ice cream

SEX SCRAMBLE

Do you know the names of these sex toys and accessories?
Unscramble the anagrams.

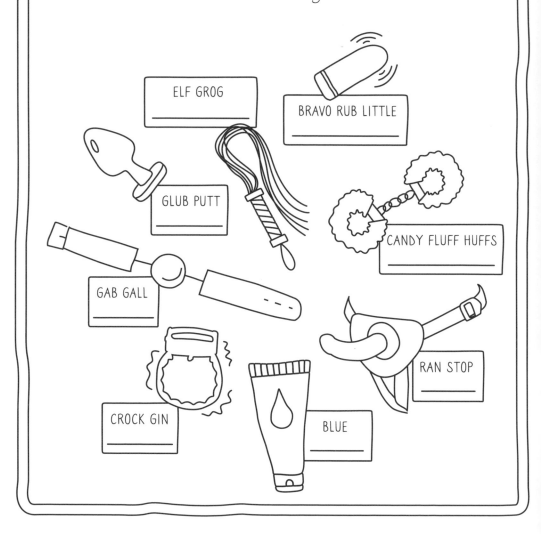

ELF GROG
_____

BRAVO RUB LITTLE
_____

GLUB PUTT
_____

CANDY FLUFF HUFFS
_____

GAB GALL
_____

RAN STOP
_____

CROCK GIN
_____

BLUE
_____

Sex-duko

Use your arty skills and fill in the missing pictures in the grid – there must be one of each picture in each row, column and section.

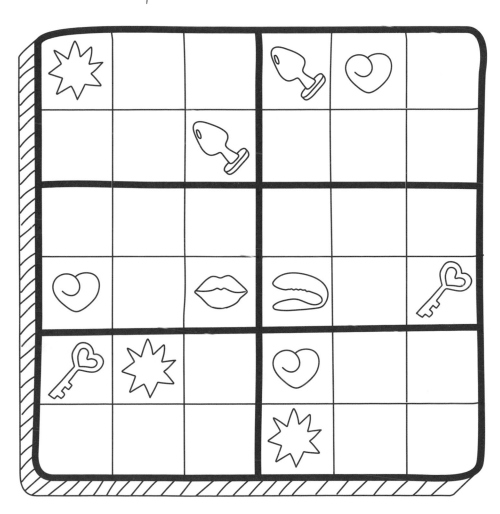

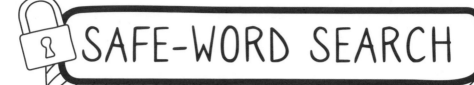

SAFE-WORD SEARCH

Everything you do together should be 100% consensual. To ensure this is the case, agree a safe word before you play. Safe words are used by either partner to indicate they want play to stop immediately. Choose a word that is easy to remember and that you wouldn't normally say when you're having a good time. Or try the popular 'traffic light' system, where 'red' means stop, 'amber' means take it easy and 'green' means go on.

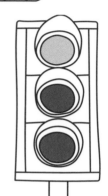

Find the safe-word suggestions in the grid.

- ☐ AMBER
- ☐ BANANA
- ☐ DONALD DUCK
- ☐ KANGAROO
- ☐ LATTE
- ☐ PEACH
- ☐ RED
- ☐ SANTA
- ☐ SHED
- ☐ SPAIN
- ☐ TEAPOT
- ☐ TULIP
- ☐ VEGETABLES
- ☐ VODKA

B	E	K	S	S	A	N	T	A	N
V	H	C	A	E	P	X	O	T	I
D	O	U	S	P	Z	A	O	O	A
E	W	D	S	J	N	O	W	P	P
H	R	D	K	B	R	N	Y	A	S
S	E	L	B	A	T	E	G	E	V
A	B	A	G	N	U	X	D	T	O
O	M	N	E	A	L	R	T	T	S
E	A	O	T	N	I	G	E	A	T
K	M	D	T	A	P	S	H	L	S

Now finish off this bondage fantasy sketch

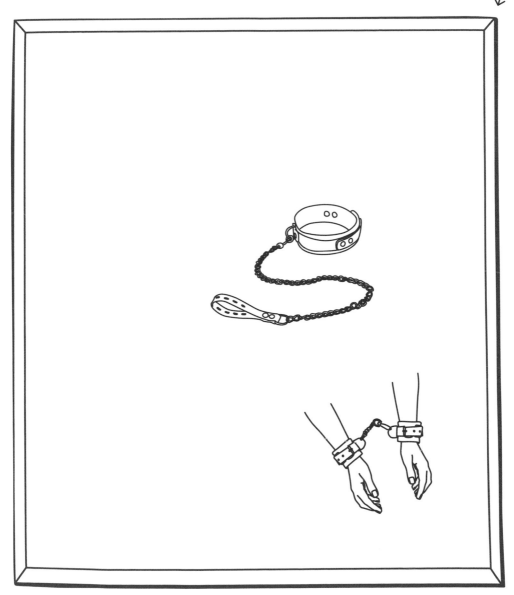

Sex Sketching

Draw your ideal sexual activity on this page.
Then ask your partner to draw theirs on the opposite page.
How do they compare? Maybe you should try them both out....

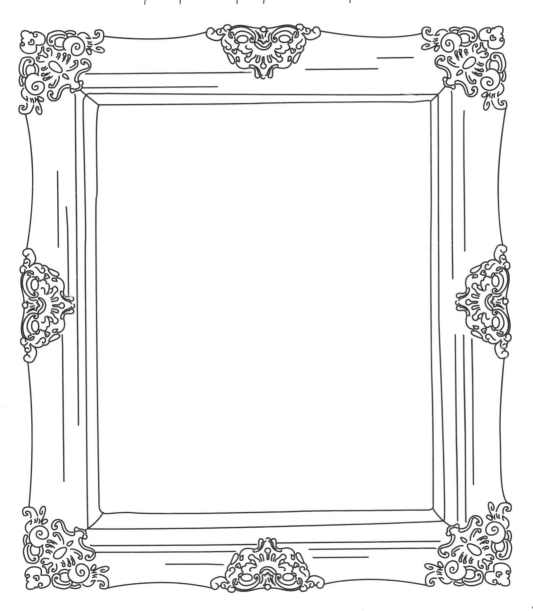

MAZE OF MASTURBATION

Can you find the path to pleasure through this maze?

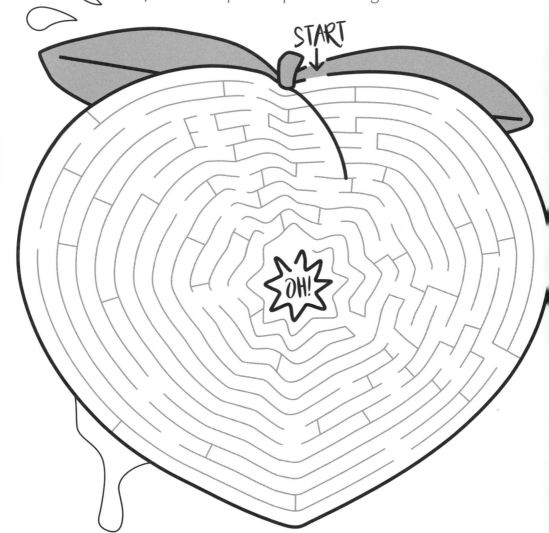

SEXUAL TOKENS

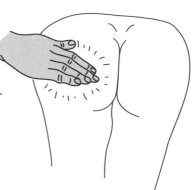

Cut out and give these tokens to your partner. Tell them they can use one per week at any time they choose, and you'll complete the activity on the token within 24 hours...

1 x ORAL SEX SESSION

This token entitles the holder to receive one session of oral sex lasting 30 minutes or until climax — whichever comes first.

1 x BONDAGE SESSION

This token entitles the holder to receive one bondage sex session, either as the dominant or submissive partner — you choose.

1 x SENSUAL MASSAGE

This token entitles the holder to receive one sensual massage lasting 30 minutes.

1 x ROLE-PLAY SESSION

This token entitles the holder to receive one role-play session, with a scenario of their choosing.

1 x HOT DATE

This token entitles the holder to receive one hot date — a meal, a few drinks, and anything else they fancy...

1 x PAMPER DAY

This token entitles the holder to receive one day (and evening) of total pampering — a foot rub, a cuddle, a bubble bath... and anything else the holder chooses.

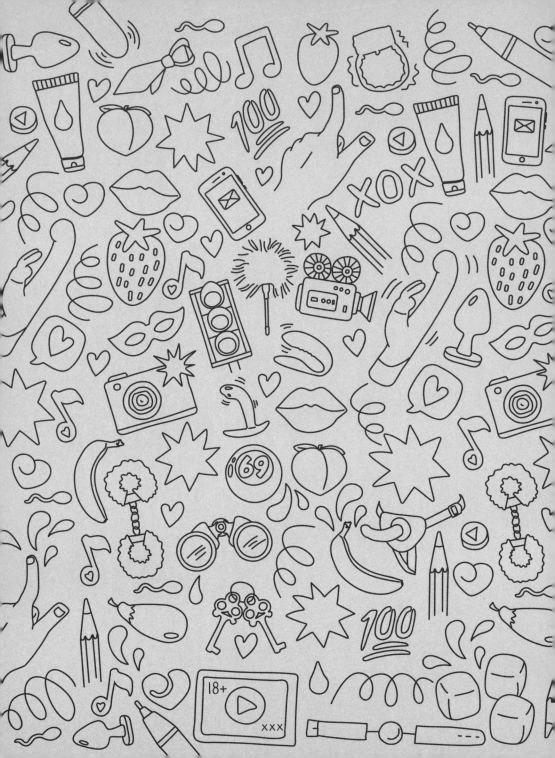

CLUE ME UP

Can you answer the clues to fill the grid?

ACROSS

2. A sphere that goes in the mouth to stop someone speaking or moving their tongue. (4,3)
4. The short name for a woman's most sensitive sexual part. (4)
6. The name of a whip with several fronds. (7)
8. A group of people engaging in sexual fun together. (4)
9. The fun that often (but not always) happens before penetration. (8)
11. The common name for a mini vibrator. (6)
13. A way of talking to get in the mood. (5)

DOWN

1. The act of pleasuring oneself. (12)
3. An agreed term a partner can say to stop proceedings. (4,4)
5. A vibrating toy that can be worn on a man's penis. (4,4)
7. Pretending to be other people along with your partner. (4,4)
10. The opening in your bottom where plugs might go. (4)
12. The act of stroking someone with a feather. (6)

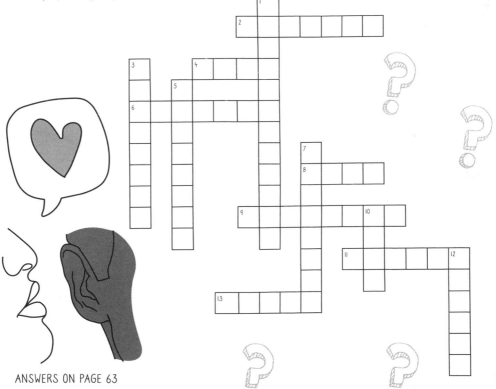

ANSWERS ON PAGE 63

Fantasy Feels

The location I want to do it in is...

because...

The character I want to be is...

because...

The character I want you to be is...

because...

Use these pages to reveal those fantasies you can't get out of your head. When you're done, show them to your partner and see what happens. If you're currently single, save them for future use!

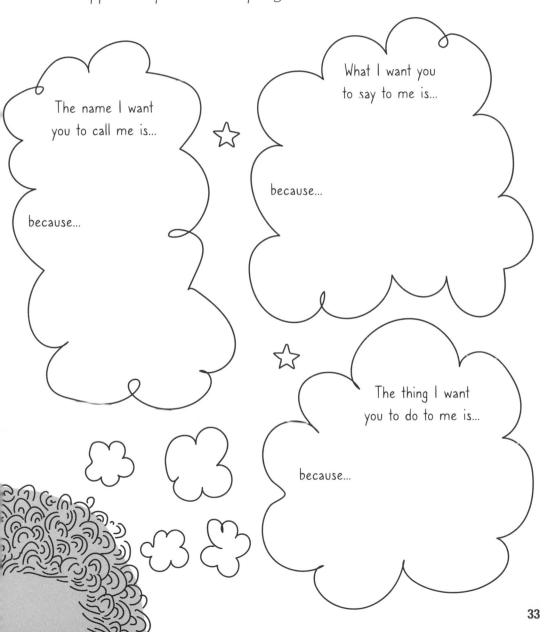

The name I want
you to call me is...

because...

What I want you
to say to me is...

because...

The thing I want
you to do to me is...

because...

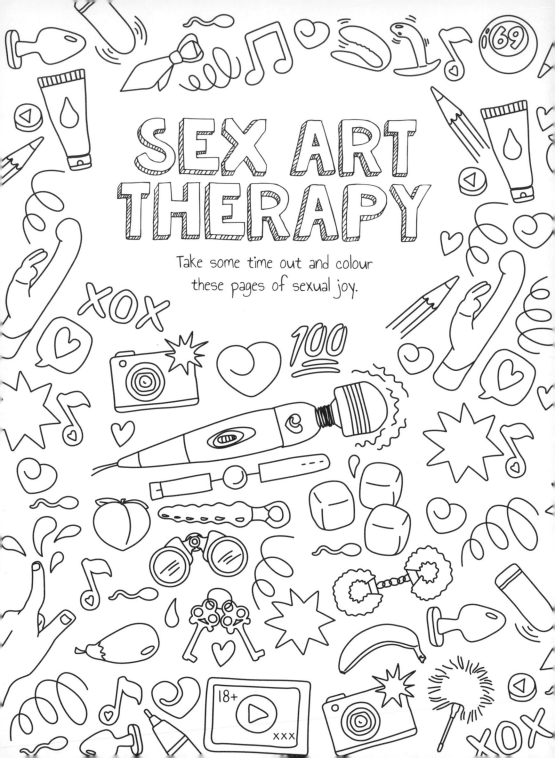

SEX ART THERAPY

Take some time out and colour
these pages of sexual joy.

WOULD YOU RATHER...?

Answer these questions by putting a tick next to the ones you'd rather do. Then ask your partner to add their own ticks in a different colour. How do things match up? If you have different preferences... why not try everything?

Would you rather...

Be dominant in the bedroom **OR** Be submissive in the bedroom

Watch an adult movie together **OR** Read an erotic novel to each other

Watch another couple having sex **OR** Let someone watch you have sex

Give oral sex **OR** Receive oral sex

Give up masturbation **OR** Never receive oral sex again

Talk dirty over the phone **OR** Talk dirty through text messages

Have sex in the morning **OR** Have sex at night

Be spanked **OR** Receive a sexy massage

☐ ☐   ☐ ☐

Be gagged **OR** Be blindfolded

☐ ☐   ☐ ☐

Watch your partner masturbate **OR** Be watched by your partner

☐ ☐   ☐ ☐

Slow and sensual **OR** Hard and fast

☐ ☐   ☐ ☐

Lights on **OR** Lights off

☐ ☐   ☐ ☐

Use sex toys **OR** Use fingers

☐ ☐   ☐ ☐

Come first **OR** Come second

☐ ☐   ☐ ☐

Loud sex in an empty house **OR** Quiet sex because other people are in

☐ ☐   ☐ ☐

Be told what to do **OR** Tell your partner what to do

☐ ☐   ☐ ☐

Spank your partner **OR** Get spanked

☐ ☐   ☐ ☐

Have sex on a plane **OR** Have sex in your office

☐ ☐   ☐ ☐

DOT-TO-HOT

Complete these dot-to-dots to reveal
two hot sexual positions and their names.

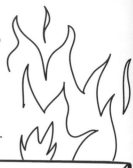

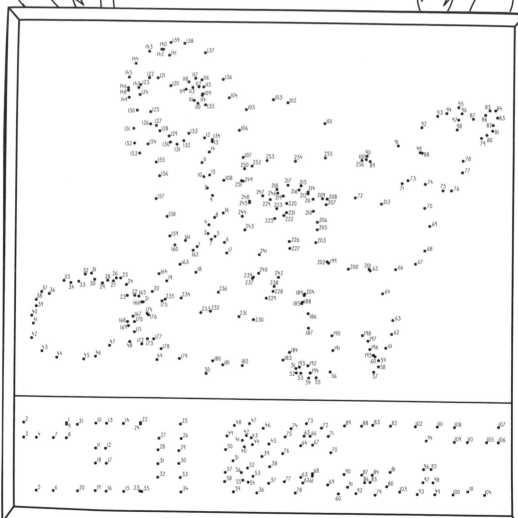

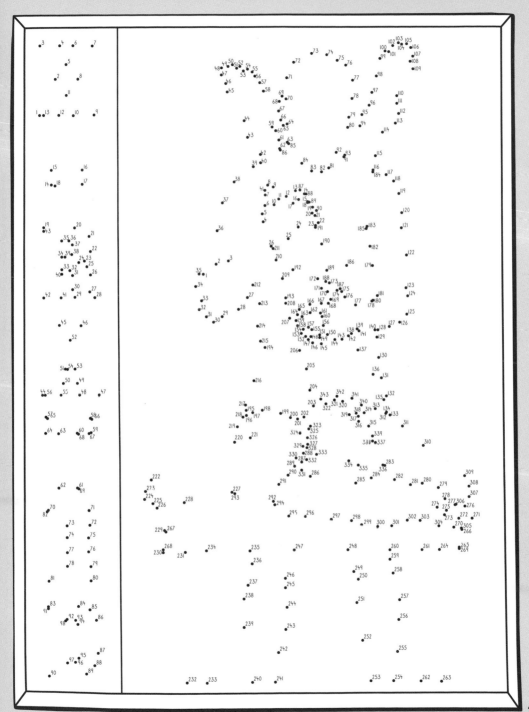

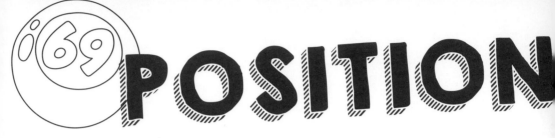

69 POSITION

Complete the positions on the grids with your partner to make as many full horizontal, vertical or diagonal lines as you can. Bingoooooooh!

BACKWARDS COWGIRL	GIDDY-UP	THIGH MASTER	TIP-TO-TOE	BOTTOMS UP 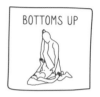
STANDING THRUST	RAUNCHY RIDER	THE MISSIONARY	FACE-TO-FACE	UP AGAINST IT 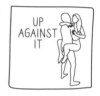
JOINED AT THE HIP	VOYEUR'S DELIGHT	GIRL POWER	HAND IT TO HIM	TIGHT SQUEEZE
THE BABE BENDOVER	THE SANDWICH	THE COVER-UP	THE LEG LIFT	DOGGY ON THE BED 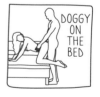
SEXY SPOON 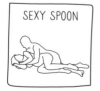	THE DANCER	SIT-DOWN SEX	OPEN SESAME	ROCK CHICK

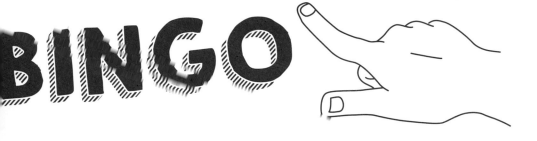

BINGO

LAZY LEG-OVER	SEXY YOGA	THE PROPOSAL	HORSING AROUND 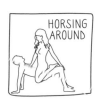	FLYING HIGH
THE GRIND	X-RATED	HOT SEAT 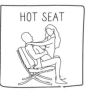	ROCK AND LOCK	CROSSED LOVERS
THE CAN-CAN	MISSION IMPOSSIBLE	LUSTY LEAN	THE SQUAT	THE LOVE SEAT
DOGGY STYLE	HEAD OVER HEELS	THE WATERFALL	FISHBONE	STAND AND DELIVER
THE SEE-SAW	TABLE TOP	CLOSE ENCOUNTER	THE CORKSCREW	THE PUMP

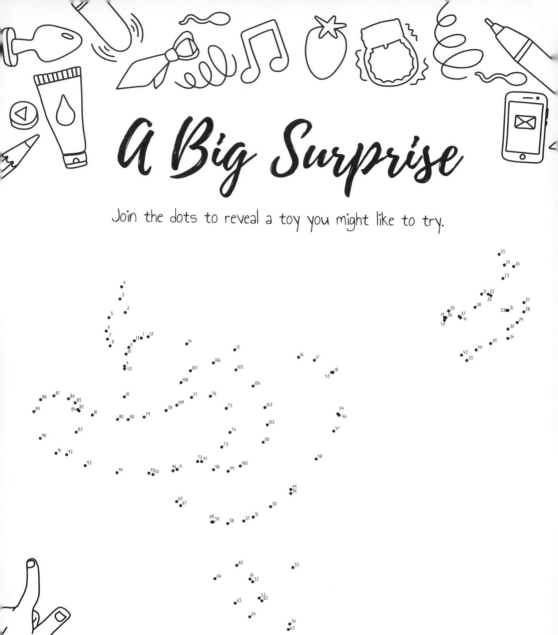

A Big Surprise

Join the dots to reveal a toy you might like to try.

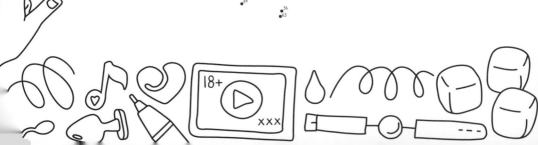

KISS-CROSS

Fill the words into the grid with only their length as a clue. Size matters - but only for this puzzle.

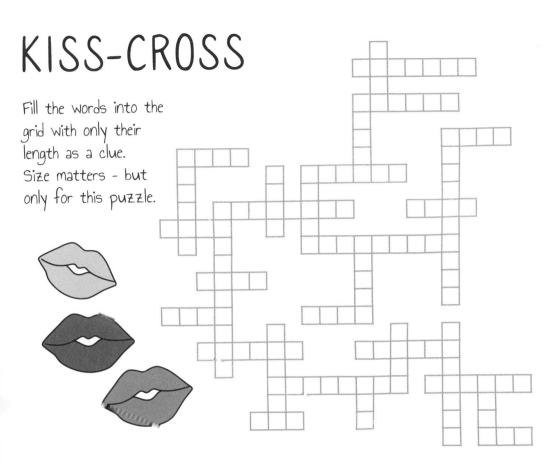

3 LETTERS
ASK
BEG
SEX

4 LETTERS
ANUS
COME
DATE
KISS
LICK
LOVE

4 LETTERS CONT...
PLAY
SAFE
SEXY
TEXT
WHIP

5 LETTERS
DIRTY
SPANK
TOUCH

6 LETTERS
CLIMAX
CUDDLE
ORGASM
PLEASE
SECRET
TICKLE
TONGUE

7 LETTERS
BEDROOM
BONDAGE

8 LETTERS
DOMINANT
PLEASURE

9 LETTERS
HANDCUFFS

10 LETTERS
PERMISSION
SUBMISSIVE

ANSWERS ON PAGE 63

FIND THE RIGHT POSITION

- [ ] BABE BENDOVER
- [ ] BACKWARDS COWGIRL
- [ ] BOTTOMS-UP
- [ ] CAN-CAN
- [ ] CLOSE ENCOUNTER
- [ ] CORKSCREW
- [ ] COVER-UP
- [ ] CROSSED LOVERS
- [ ] DANCER
- [ ] DOGGY ON THE BED
- [ ] DOGGY STYLE
- [ ] FACE-TO-FACE
- [ ] FISHBONE
- [ ] FLYING HIGH
- [ ] GIDDY-UP
- [ ] GIRL POWER
- [ ] GRIND
- [ ] HAND IT TO HIM
- [ ] HEAD OVER HEELS
- [ ] HOLD TIGHT
- [ ] HORSING AROUND
- [ ] HOT SEAT
- [ ] JOINED AT THE HIP
- [ ] LAZY LEG-OVER
- [ ] LEG LIFT
- [ ] LOVE SEAT

B	F	H	S	Z	H	H	A	X	I	H	O	D	P	K	L	A	A	U	B	B	F	Z	G	E
R	Y	D	G	M	F	O	G	G	A	W	E	K	U	G	Z	W	E	T	A	C	U	V	W	C
Y	Y	K	L	C	M	W	R	N	L	B	U	J	R	R	S	J	S	C	B	Q	H	L	J	A
F	X	O	H	E	D	P	D	S	E	N	K	R	E	C	I	N	K	S	E	L	L	V	L	F
M	K	B	N	D	G	I	S	H	I	L	R	B	V	K	K	W	Z	R	B	S	R	X	X	O
A	W	L	G	O	T	L	T	U	G	N	N	U	O	C	A	U	U	E	E	T	F	J	G	T
T	H	G	R	T	R	N	I	K	Q	O	G	X	C	R	D	I	Z	V	N	L	J	H	I	E
E	H	Q	O	L	O	M	D	F	M	X	E	A	D	A	U	J	H	O	D	W	X	S	Y	C
E	Y	H	S	Y	P	A	Y	N	T	F	H	S	R	E	J	O	D	L	O	Y	O	J	Y	A
O	I	C	G	X	N	I	F	B	T	U	C	B	L	O	L	F	T	D	V	K	T	F	A	F
M	Z	G	B	C	T	N	H	Z	A	O	R	U	B	D	U	Y	L	E	E	X	Z	A	F	G
V	O	T	E	K	C	A	G	E	W	I	E	L	T	H	K	N	T	S	R	V	I	Q	M	I
D	G	R	A	R	K	R	E	G	H	N	J	I	C	W	O	P	D	S	M	L	Q	Y	Y	R
Z	N	E	S	I	U	C	I	S	S	T	G	Q	N	S	O	E	P	O	Y	O	G	V	U	L
T	K	K	D	R	Y	R	O	Z	E	H	T	Z	O	K	W	C	L	R	K	G	U	H	R	P
W	S	M	C	G	L	A	N	R	T	V	I	A	W	N	E	B	A	C	K	T	G	U	K	O
Q	F	K	U	A	T	V	U	S	K	Y	O	V	D	E	N	O	B	H	S	I	F	O	D	W
R	E	T	N	U	O	C	N	E	E	S	O	L	C	E	N	Z	P	N	H	B	A	C	D	E
H	O	T	S	E	A	T	P	U	J	N	C	Z	Q	V	N	U	J	G	C	B	Z	G	V	R
P	U	Y	X	J	B	S	X	S	A	E	U	R	Q	Z	Y	I	N	K	A	D	N	I	R	G
H	E	A	D	O	V	E	R	H	E	E	L	S	E	D	B	I	O	Y	N	V	U	P	S	R
R	E	V	O	G	E	L	Y	Z	A	L	X	F	D	W	Y	Y	V	J	C	D	V	P	T	Z
O	S	Q	C	L	X	W	E	Z	B	C	M	I	J	L	J	G	G	O	A	H	Y	R	Z	J
F	V	C	P	F	C	O	N	P	S	N	G	L	F	T	Q	X	X	L	N	O	N	I	T	G
U	X	B	O	T	T	O	M	S	U	P	G	E	B	A	G	I	H	M	Q	G	R	H	P	J

The names of 52 sexual positions are hidden in these two grids
(26 in each). Can you find (and then try) them all?

- ☐ LUSTY LEAN
- ☐ MISSIONARY
- ☐ MISSION IMPOSSIBLE
- ☐ OPEN SESAME
- ☐ PROPOSAL
- ☐ PUMP

- ☐ RAUNCHY RIDER
- ☐ ROCK AND LOCK
- ☐ ROCK CHICK
- ☐ SANDWICH
- ☐ SEE-SAW
- ☐ SEXY SPOON
- ☐ SEXY YOGA

- ☐ SIT-DOWN SEX
- ☐ SQUAT
- ☐ STAND AND DELIVER
- ☐ STANDING THRUST
- ☐ TABLE TOP
- ☐ THIGH MASTER

- ☐ TIGHT SQUEEZE
- ☐ TIP-TO-TOE
- ☐ UP AGAINST IT
- ☐ VOYEUR'S DELIGHT
- ☐ WATERFALL
- ☐ WHEELBARROW
- ☐ X-RATED

V	V	M	T	N	C	Q	F	M	P	K	M	B	S	U	S	E	W	E	M	F	Q	C	Z	M
I	W	L	W	B	J	C	K	X	J	P	X	B	O	N	O	W	Z	Z	I	M	D	H	F	N
Y	C	F	J	W	F	P	L	J	T	H	W	A	K	T	K	E	I	K	S	I	A	R	V	U
K	H	X	T	F	C	X	Y	L	K	M	V	Y	O	T	E	L	U	W	S	N	X	W	X	U
T	S	U	R	H	T	G	N	I	D	N	A	T	S	U	H	B	P	N	I	O	T	W	I	S
P	T	V	E	F	P	H	L	U	E	G	P	C	Q	G	U	I	A	V	O	K	K	I	F	H
X	S	P	D	W	Z	Y	G	M	C	I	B	S	W	S	M	E	G	P	N	Q	C	E	R	F
E	P	C	I	A	Q	W	S	I	T	S	T	H	T	E	L	N	A	H	I	H	Z	J	T	D
S	O	X	R	P	K	K	Q	X	L	H	E	A	N	Y	M	Y	I	O	M	X	K	O	Y	H
N	T	S	Y	R	Z	E	L	U	G	E	N	X	T	U	M	A	N	Q	P	A	S	O	V	W
W	E	S	H	Z	P	W	E	I	L	D	D	S	Y	M	W	H	S	A	O	P	S	U	C	D
O	L	D	C	W	S	W	T	B	A	I	U	S	X	S	L	Y	T	E	S	N	P	T	C	X
D	B	F	N	Y	W	E	A	N	W	L	B	Z	R	R	P	Z	I	H	S	M	P	S	E	X
T	A	P	U	U	S	R	D	D	F	C	J	P	X	U	A	O	T	Z	I	N	E	E	I	R
I	T	O	A	L	R	D	H	C	I	W	D	N	A	S	E	T	O	O	B	T	E	V	A	W
S	V	F	R	O	E	R	O	C	K	C	H	I	C	K	Z	Y	E	N	L	G	M	P	L	A
Q	W	G	W	L	T	G	Z	M	P	T	J	J	L	O	B	D	O	D	E	T	X	M	O	T
U	X	K	I	J	B	Q	G	R	A	A	Y	U	T	Z	B	P	A	V	K	H	Q	C	S	E
A	R	V	R	O	A	G	O	T	Z	U	G	V	N	J	X	E	U	A	T	I	J	J	U	R
T	E	J	D	N	C	P	G	K	L	M	R	O	C	K	A	N	D	L	O	C	K	V	L	F
R	Y	R	A	N	O	I	S	S	I	M	P	B	Y	Q	N	I	Y	N	P	C	X	E	J	A
Y	D	N	F	S	V	M	U	X	K	U	U	T	K	Y	S	E	E	S	A	W	A	Y	O	L
O	B	P	A	Q	L	L	R	X	M	O	R	R	F	Q	X	O	S	C	L	Z	E	S	X	L
D	I	L	X	P	K	Q	X	P	H	Q	N	V	V	F	N	E	U	I	V	K	Y	P	G	V
A	R	I	Y	B	U	K	M	H	O	W	D	L	E	A	V	B	S	H	B	U	H	T	N	F

Love Letters

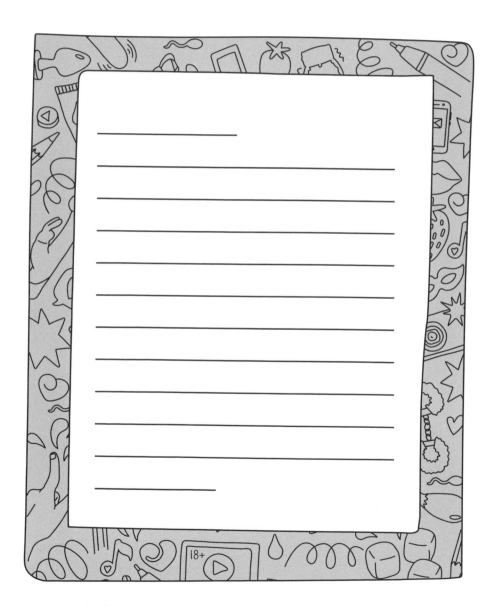

Use this page to write a sexy love letter to your partner - telling them all the things you love about your sex life, and a few things you'd like to try. Ask your partner to write their reply on the opposite page...

18+

WHAT TYPE OF LOVER ARE YOU?

Answer yes or no to each statement to reveal which type of lover you are. It's just for fun... but might reveal something you didn't know about yourself.

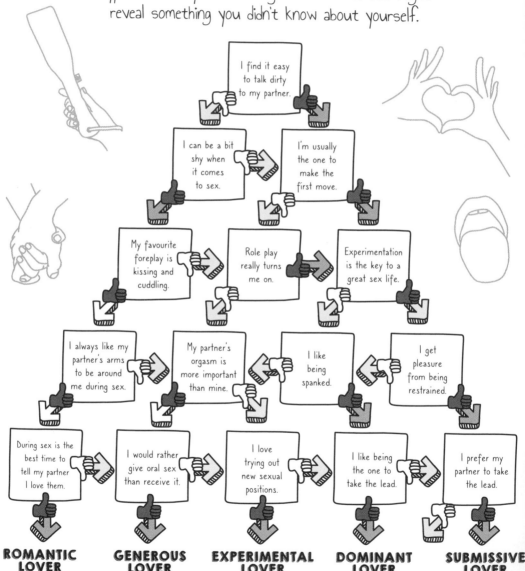

I find it easy to talk dirty to my partner.

I can be a bit shy when it comes to sex.

I'm usually the one to make the first move.

My favourite foreplay is kissing and cuddling.

Role play really turns me on.

Experimentation is the key to a great sex life.

I always like my partner's arms to be around me during sex.

My partner's orgasm is more important than mine.

I like being spanked.

I get pleasure from being restrained.

During sex is the best time to tell my partner I love them.

I would rather give oral sex than receive it.

I love trying out new sexual positions.

I like being the one to take the lead.

I prefer my partner to take the lead.

ROMANTIC LOVER

GENEROUS LOVER

EXPERIMENTAL LOVER

DOMINANT LOVER

SUBMISSIVE LOVER

ROMANTIC LOVER

For you, sex is all about expressing your deep love for your partner.
You like to kiss and cuddle, look each other in the eyes, and make slow, sensual love.
Nothing turns you on more than a romantic evening ending up in a warm, cosy bed.

GENEROUS LOVER

You like to focus on your partner's pleasure before thinking about your own.
You love giving oral sex or pleasing your partner with your hands.
Seeing them enjoying themselves really turns you on.

EXPERIMENTAL LOVER

For you, the key to a great sex life is variation.
You love trying different positions, role-play scenarios, locations and sex toys.
You get turned on by things you haven't done before.

DOMINANT LOVER

You're the type of lover who likes to be in charge.
You love to restrain, spank and tease your partner — and tell them what to do.
You get turned on by taking the lead.

SUBMISSIVE LOVER

You love being with a partner who takes control.
You might spend the rest of your life making decisions, but during sex, you like to let go.
You love being restrained, spanked and given instructions by your partner.

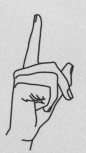

REMEMBER...

Whichever result you got, this doesn't mean you don't like to go outside your comfort zone from time to time. Ask your partner to complete the quiz, too, and it might help you understand each other's desires - and decide to try something different in the bedroom!

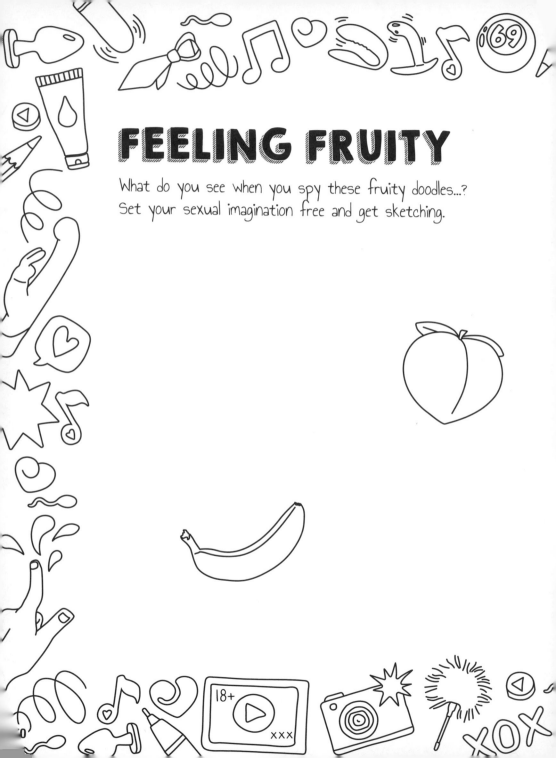

FEELING FRUITY

What do you see when you spy these fruity doodles...?
Set your sexual imagination free and get sketching.

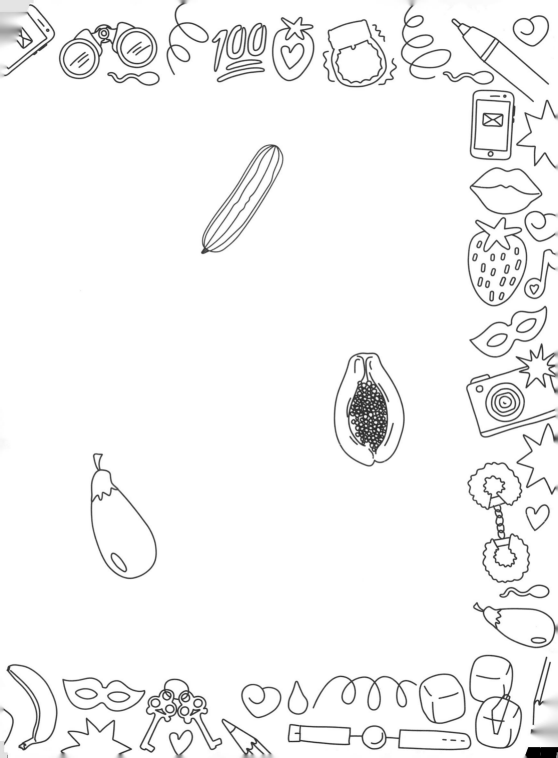

Raunchy Route

Follow the key to find the right route through the grid.

START

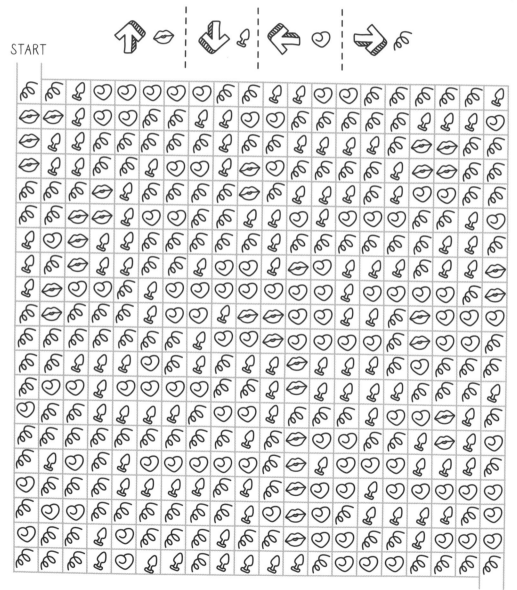

FINISH

COME AND COLOUR

Colour and decorate these sex toys any way you choose.

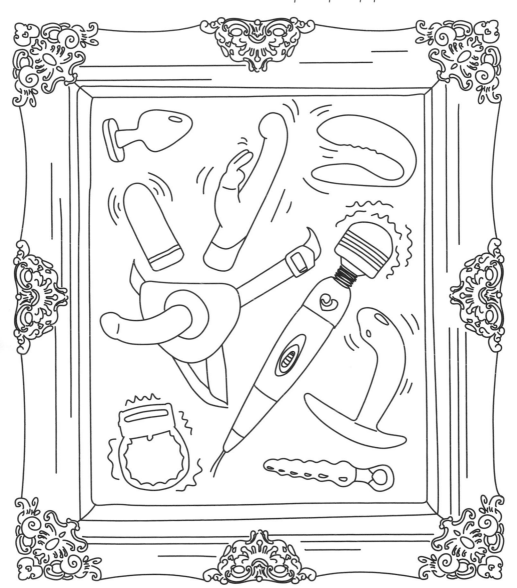

FILL ME IN

Fill in the blanks of this sexy message
sent from one partner to another.

I've been thinking about you all day,

especially your _____ .

I can't wait for you to get home so

I can _____ your _____ .

I'm going to ask you to _____

my _____ until I _____ .

When you touch my _____ it

makes me feel _____ , and I want

you to do it tonight. After that, I want to

watch you _____ .

I want to make you come _____ times.

First I'll use _____ , then I'll

use _____ _____ and _____ .

I want you to _____ _____ me.

One day I'd love it if we can go to

_____ and _____

while nobody is around. I want you to

call me _____ . Let's pretend to be

a _____ , and a _____

while we pleasure each other.

Something I've always wanted to try is

_____ .

Will you try it with me...?

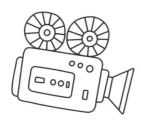

Word Play

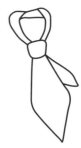

Each answer in this crossword is the name of a role you might play in a sexy fantasy scenario. Can you crack the clues?

ACROSS

2. You might have to show them the ways of this planet. (5)
7. You just write each other sexy letters. (3,6)
8. Someone who might keep you hostage on their ship. (6)
9. Hopefully they'll bring you more than your food. (6)
10. Someone delivering a package. (8,6)
13. Someone who will send your pleasure sky-high. (5)
14. They might take you to a show, and the after-party... (4,4)
18. They'll want to take your picture. (12)
19. Someone who's being taught something. (7)
20. You'll have to pay them for their services. (6)

DOWN

1. You'll definitely need mouth-to-mouth from this person. (4,5)
3. A person that likes to watch. (6)
4. They only come out at night. (7)
5. Someone lending you more than just books. (9)
6. Someone doing a job at a desk. (6,6)
11. You might have seen them in a few x-rated movies. (4,4)
12. Remember to bow or curtsey to them. (7)
15. They'll whip you up something delicious. (4)
16. You'll have to programme them to obey you. (5)
17. They'll give you a thorough examination. (6)

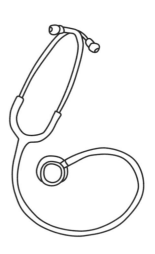

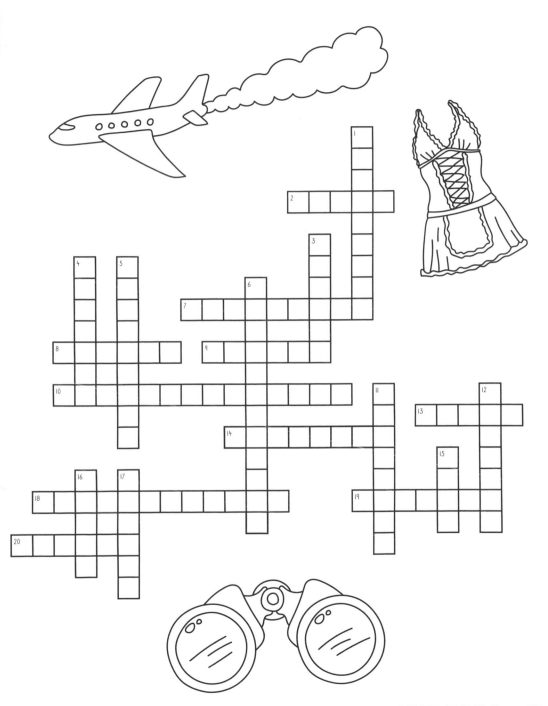

Sex Planner

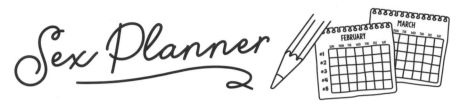

It might surprise you to hear that forward-planning is one of the best ways to improve the sex life in a relationship. Along with your partner, use these pages to jot down some pleasure plans for the next few weeks. Include new things to try - role-play scenarios, sex-toy suggestions, positions and more! Afterwards, make some notes on things you enjoyed and why.

DATE:

Pleasure plan:

How was it for you?

DATE:

Pleasure plan:

How was it for you?

DATE:

Pleasure plan:

How was it for you?

DATE:

Pleasure plan:

How was it for you?

DATE:

Pleasure plan:

How was it for you?

DATE:

Pleasure plan:

How was it for you?

DATE:

Pleasure plan:

How was it for you?

DATE:

Pleasure plan:

How was it for you?

DATE:

Pleasure plan:

How was it for you?

DATE:

Pleasure plan:

How was it for you?

DATE:

Pleasure plan:

How was it for you?

ANSWERS

PAGE 6
SEARCH FOR SATISFACTION

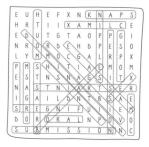

PAGES 12-13
DIRTY SECRETS

1. I WANT TO TASTE YOU
2. WHERE DO YOU WANT ME TO COME
3. I WANT TO HEAR YOU BEG
4. GET ON YOUR KNEES
5. BEND OVER I AM GOING TO SPANK YOU
6. WATCH WHILE I TOUCH MYSELF
7. I WANT YOU TO F*CK MY MOUTH
8. ARE YOU READY TO COME AGAIN FOR ME
9. LET'S WATCH PORN TOGETHER
10. YOU LOOK SEXY WHEN YOU GO DOWN ON ME

PAGE 23
SEX-DUKO

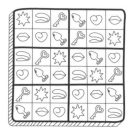

PAGE 8
G-SPOT THE DIFFERENCE

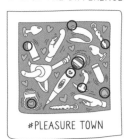

#PLEASURE TOWN

PAGES 18-19
HOT WORD CROSSWORD

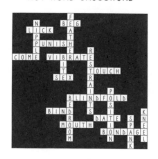

PAGES 24-25
SAFE-WORD SEARCH

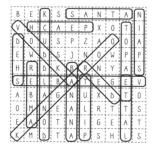

PAGE 11
I'M HARD

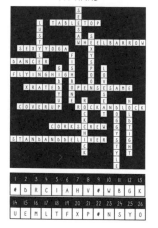

PAGE 22
SEX SCRAMBLE

ELF GROG - FLOGGER
BRAVO RUB LITTLE - BULLET VIBRATOR
GLUB PUTT - BUTT PLUG
CANDY FLUFF HUFFS - FLUFFY HANDCUFFS
GAB GALL - BALL GAG
RAN STOP - STRAP ON
CROCK GIN - COCK RING
BLUE - LUBE

PAGE 28
MAZE OF MASTURBATION

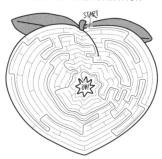

PAGE 31
CLUE ME UP

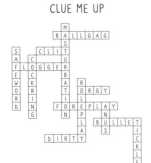

PAGES 38-39
DOT-TO-HOT

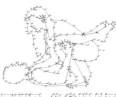

PAGE 42
A BIG SURPRISE

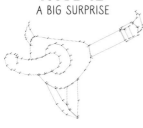

PAGE 43
KISS-CROSS

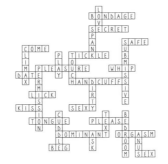

PAGES 44-45
FIND THE RIGHT POSITION

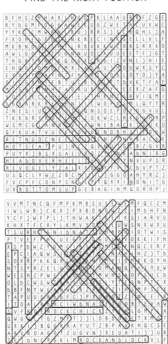

PAGE 52
RAUNCHY ROUTE

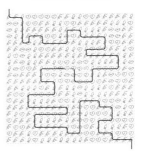

PAGES 56-57
WORD PLAY

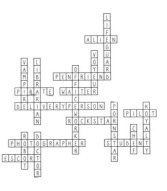

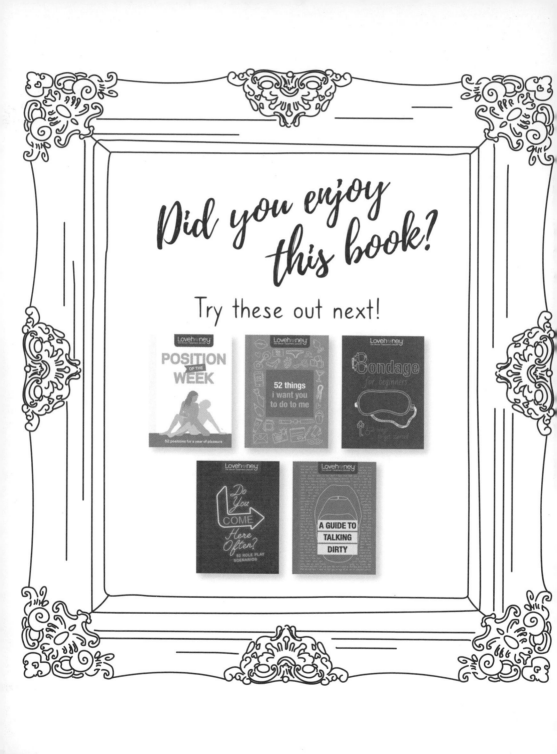